STOP SMOKING
The Hard Way

If One of the Easy Ways Had Worked
You Wouldn't Be Reading This

Scott Lee

Contents

Schoolhouse Earth Volumes are basically the same. That is because I believe Spiritual Practices like these are necessary to any successful life endeavor.

SMOKING CESSATION PROGRAM

INTRODUCTION

In the summer of 1985 I realized that smoking cigarettes was in violation of the spiritual principles I was trying to live by. A friend told me that he had tried a new smoking cessation program that worked for him. The following is only partially that program. I have added quite a bit and most of my additions are of a spiritual nature.

Smoking is an addiction but it is also a habit. My analysis is that the following program slowly removes the habit first. When the habit is defeated it is then much easier to overcome the addiction.

My experience is that patches and nicotine gum just seem to prolong the inevitable withdrawal time from the addiction and only offer limited help with the habit.

You can try this program alone or with one or more others who really want to quit. This program has worked for many folks who used it by themselves. I strongly recommend that you form a group if at all possible because of the mutual support. If you opt for a group I suggest you assemble as many as 10 people who are deadly serious about quitting. Ask everyone who wants to be in the group to read the entire program before the first meeting. Those who say they will read it but don't will probably drop of your group soon after you start. Those who are at least committed enough to read all of this in the period before the first meeting are probably dedicated enough to go through it with you.

Nicotine is a serious addiction. It is not easy to stop or many, many people would have already stopped and you are probably one of them or you wouldn't be reading this right now. Because it is so addictive, overcoming nicotine addiction requires a serious effort over a considerable period of time.

It involves much more than quitting. It really requires a major life-style change.

Schedule your meeting for 1 hour. Usually 7 or 7:30 PM is a good start time. Good meetings start on time. Great meetings end on time. Do not delay your opening for any tardy members. If you do delay for them you will eventually lose some of those who are punctual.

Don't allow your meeting to run late. If you do, some of your married members will soon drop out.

The meeting is obviously tobacco free.

NOTE: The term "cigarette" is used generically throughout this document. It means whatever form of tobacco the person is using. It could be cigarettes, cigarillos, cigars, snuff, pipes, etc.

Session I

GETTING STARTED

Open your meeting with a prayer. Any prayer will do for the first session and silent prayer might be best to begin with. This is a spiritual approach to smoking cessation. Don't be bashful about prayer.

In Session I each "quitter" will discuss his/her reasons for wanting to quit as well as talking about other methods they have tried to get off of nicotine. They will also tell the group how many cigarettes they estimate they smoked per day last week.

Each then verbally commits to the group to go to any length to complete the entire process. This includes participation and early arrival at ALL meetings and "doing the 'do's" and not "doing the don'ts". It also means committing to 45 minutes per day, 6 days each week, to homework assignments, meditation, exercise, etc. This is a massive commitment. Everyone needs to understand and agree to it. There is also a commitment to 2 hours for 1 day per week on meeting day. These 2 hours include travel time.

Each "quitter" agrees **NOT TO TELL ANYONE** except their spouse about this program. They also commit not to discuss quitting or this program with anyone except group members and those discussions will be limited to **during meetings only!** This means not discussing this subject with members of the group outside of these meetings. Please don't drain the energy you have for this process in the form of loose talk; and don't bleed off the energy from your group meetings by discussing this with group members outside of the meetings.

The group selects a group name and decides on the opening/closing prayers and ceremonies. Some effective prayers for opening are: The Saint Francis Prayer and The Serenity Prayer. Either of these two or The Lord's Prayer are all good selections for closing.

Some name suggestions are: Quitters, Lungers, Clean Air Group, Healthys.

The Opening/Closing Ceremony is typically something like a few moments of silence followed by the selected prayer followed by three hard, deep breaths followed by about 5 minutes of meditation. There are many books on meditation. Ask each member to buy one and rotate leading this 5 minute beginning meditation. After the meditation the leader will lead the group in a slow, deep breath followed by an audible sigh.

The group leader passes out golf pencils, rubber bands and slips of paper approximately the size of a cigarette pack and explains the "log it or skip it" program.

Log It or Skip It: Each member will now wrap the paper around his/her pack and use the rubber band to secure the paper and the golf pencil to the pack. For the next week each quitter will "log" each cigarette by time of day and current activity. What time was it and what were you doing when you decided to have this cigarette?

Your log will look something like this:

Monday, 4-9-2012

7:15AM after breakfast

8:05 driving to work

9:15 coffee break

10:00 at desk

10:45 getting coffee

11:30 in the car going to lunch

12:35 after lunch

12:38 after lunch

12:55 going back to work

Etc.

If someone asks you about the log, DO NOT MENTION THAT YOU ARE QUITTING! Tell him you are just looking at your smoking habit and change the subject. YOU DON'T WANT TO TALK ABOUT IT!

Cut additional sheets of paper to fit your pack and use a new one each day. Put the day and date at the top of each sheet and save them throughout the entire process. You will want to review them at later sessions to help you understand your smoking patterns.

From this meeting on, NO carton purchases. NO 100mm, king size or other longer than normal cigarettes may be purchased or smoked. No bumming smokes from others. No nicotine gum, patches, etc. Continue to smoke your normal brand.

You may not add the use of other types of tobacco such as snuff, chewing tobacco, cigars, etc. You may continue to use them if they have been part of your daily nicotine consumption. If this is the case, you must "log or skip" as with cigarettes.

Each group member commits to attending ALL meetings and to doing a minimum of fifteen minutes of meditation at a specific time each day for the next 10 weeks. Each member tells the group when his meditations will be until the next meeting. Participants may change their time of day on meditation as they wish at the meeting but not between meetings. Some will select early morning, others evening but it is imperative that each one commits to a specific time.

HOMEWORK: Each quitter writes a brief paragraph on why she started smoking, why she is quitting, and how badly she wants to quit. Also, look up and write down the definitions of "habit" and "addiction" from a dictionary. Please do these before the next meeting. Do them TODAY if you're really serious about quitting.

Each member writes his/her own morning and evening prayer. The morning prayer needs to contain the request for God's help in following all of the directions just for today. The evening prayer needs to contain a thank you for the help in staying on course with this program today. If you want God to help you with this, you need to treat Him like He is real.

These prayers must be prayed daily.

Before the next meeting read the chapter earlier in this book entitled "Priorities" and do the exercise it describes. Bring your notes on this exercise to the next meeting.

Our quit date is four weeks from today.

BABY ELEPHANTS

My friend Howard loves to tell the story of a short subject movie he saw as a child. It concerned the training of baby elephants.

They began the training by securing the baby elephant's foreleg to a big stake that had been driven into the ground with a very thick rope. The baby elephant would tug and tug on the rope trying to free itself. The elephant usually struggled to free himself for a long time.

Eventually the animal would learn that no amount of tugging could free it. This could take several days. At this point the baby elephant would cease all struggling against the rope. He had finally learned that it was impossible for him to move when his foreleg was tied to a stake. The trainer would allow him to remain tied there for a while and then would untie the elephant and continue the training.

For the rest of the elephant's life the trainer could drive a relatively small stake into the ground and secure the full grown elephant's foreleg to the stake with a relatively small rope and the elephant would not struggle against the rope at all.

The same elephant had been pushing over trees in the jungle all day and dragging them out. It had plenty of strength to break the rope or to pull up the stake but it remained docilely tied up. It was not the stake that held the elephant. It was not the rope that held the elephant. It was not the combination of the stake and rope that held him.

It was his "baby elephant belief" that held the full grown elephant.

We all have "baby elephant beliefs" that hold us back if we don't learn to change them.

Here are some old baby elephant belief's I used to have. Please see if any of them are holding you back.

When you were about 7 years old weren't you certain that if you could get a bicycle you would be happy. Did you get a bike? Are you happy?

Was there a time in your life when you wanted him or her and you were certain if you could just get him/her you'd be happy? Did you get him/her? Are you happy?

Was there at time when you were certain that if you could only get rid of him/her you'd be happy? Was there? Did you get rid of them? Are you happy?

My overwhelming baby elephant belief was that if I could get what I wanted I would be happy. Not true! I was wrong about that.

I thought there was something out there that I could acquire, achieve or attain that would bring me happiness. The problem was that no matter what I got the shine always wore off.

I had happiness confused with pleasure. There are things out there on the physical plane that will bring me pleasure for a limited time but none of them will bring me happiness. Happiness isn't on the physical plane it is on the spiritual plane and the only way I can have it is to have a healthy relationship with God and with all of you. To do that, I must try to be of service to you and to God.

My point is that the beginning of learning is the realization that I do not know it all and, more importantly, that some of what I know for sure is actually wrong. I must release my grip on what I'm sure I know if I am to learn what I don't know.

SCHOOLHOUSE EARTH

I am convinced that Earth is merely a school. Based on my rather inauspicious start, I suspect I got here either by flunking out of somewhere else or by being expelled for bad behavior. I wonder if I'm not here to decide if I want to be a citizen of Heaven or maybe even to audition for a slot there.

For a guy like me the first lesson is: what does it really look like when I am running wide open trying to get the things I think I want? I am a slow learner as it took me over 40 years to begin to see the real answer to that question. The answer is that my will produces Hell and devastation in my life and the lives of my loved ones. His Will for my life provides me with everything I ever need and gifts beyond anything I could have ever imagined.

It is only after this first lesson is in place that I can begin to learn anything else. The next lesson is that much of what I think I have already learned turns out to be at best flawed and in many cases exactly wrong.

It is only after these two are firmly in place that I am initially willing and later eager to have God's Will in my life instead of my own. It is from this perspective that I am okay with signing the bottom of the blank sheet of the rest of my life and holding it up to Him and saying, "I would like for You to have Your Will in my life. I don't know what Your Will is but it has got to be better than mine. I don't have any questions about Your Plan for me and I will try not to make any suggestions to You about it from this moment on. I am volunteering to be in Your Service."

To start living on a spiritual basis I first had to develop spiritual practices to get me moving in the right direction. The following are some of the things I have learned to do to keep me on the spiritual path.

One of my mentors says that the measure of my spirituality is not whether I get off of the path; we all get off of the path. The measure is how quickly I get back on.

It is my prayer that these will help you as they have helped me.

PRIORITIES

The following exercise includes a list of things which may be priorities in your life. They are presented in no particular order. Please put these in your own personal priority order. Please add any items which are priorities to you but are not listed and delete any that do not apply to you.

Job, spouse (or girlfriend/boyfriend), religion, children, grandchildren, furthering your education, golf, fishing, gardening, money, retirement, prayer, meditation, toys (boats, airplanes, motorcycles etc), creating (writing a novel or poetry, painting, sculpting, working stained glass, pottery, etc), a vacation home, a special trip or purchase like a new car, watch TV, go to a movie, shop for groceries, reading the paper and watching the news, sleeping, eating, etc.

Please stop here and actually take out a piece of paper and pen and list these in the order of their importance in your life. There are no right or wrong orders. We are just taking inventory. Please take a few minutes and do this before you read any further.

Did you do it? Are you trying to get the most you can from this book? Then please do yourself a favor and don't proceed until you have written your priorities down in order.

Thank you for participating!

Now place a number in the margin next to each entry

corresponding to the amount of time you spent last week on the activity. Add activities such as commute to work, air travel etc. as necessary to fill out your week. The total of the numbers in your margin should be 168 as that is the number of hours in a week.

On a separate sheet of paper list these items in descending order by the time they were given last week with the biggest number first and compare this to your original list. Surprised?

How well do your lists match up? Are there items you said were important that received little or no time last week? Are you spending an inordinate amount of time on things that you are telling yourself are not important? What changes do you need to make to help your lists match up?

I hope you will spend some time analyzing and making changes.

I have discovered that my priorities are not what I say they are. My priorities are what I do. To find out what they are I don't listen to my words about the future; I inventory my actions in the recent past. Whatever was accomplished was a priority. Whatever was not accomplished was not a priority and anything I am saying to myself to the contrary is a lie that I am telling me.

I first ran across this concept in about 1989 and it made me very unhappy. I was telling myself that a number of things were priorities but I wasn't doing anything about them.

Seneca who lived from 3 BC to 65 AD said, "We should every night call ourselves to an account: What infirmity have I mastered today? What passions opposed? What temptation resisted? What virtue acquired? Our vices will abate of themselves if they be brought every day to the shrift."

It is critically important for me to examine myself daily by reviewing, in God's Presence, my actions throughout the day. What were my priorities…really?

SPREAD JOY

I first acquired a Spiritual Advisor about 27 years ago. It was a very good thing for me. I hold myself accountable to him. He knows all of my secrets and I have followed his advice with much success. I have had several Spiritual Advisors over the years. Here is some of their wisdom.

Spread joy. Find ways daily to share happiness. You can't keep happiness if you don't give it away. Plus, if I spend my day sloshing joy on others there is no way to keep it from splattering onto me. Here are some of the ways I try to spread joy:

I pray each morning to treasure my spouse and that I might not miss any opportunities to serve her today.

I smile as much as I possibly can.

I'm playful in crowds, especially in elevators and in long lines. I can lighten the burdens of others if I will stay alert for ways to do so.

I say thank you as much as I can. Sometimes I am able to see someone's whole face change when I thank them. We all need to be appreciated. I especially like to thank folks who are working when I am not. The following story is how I finally got this lesson.

As I walk the spiritual path, lessons appear at unexpected times. Several years ago we ran out of milk at noon on Christmas Day so, …….at half-time, I ran out to the car, raced down to the convenience store, rushed back to the cooler and grabbed a gallon of milk.

As I hustled up to the counter I received a gift. The gift was that I saw a human standing behind the counter on Christmas Day, probably working for minimum wage time and a half. I can't explain this very well but my heart opened up to him and said out loud, "Thanks for working on Christmas Day. I bet there is somewhere you'd rather be but, you see, my family ran out of milk and if you hadn't come in today we couldn't have gotten it. Thank you for working on Christmas Day."

He and I both cried as I said this. I'm not sure what the other folks in line behind me thought but I was so glad I spotted one of The Master's Kids who deserved to be thanked and was able to thank him.

These days I travel a lot on weekends. I am careful to express thanks to restaurant and airline employees for their weekend work. Sometimes I don't think they even notice that I said it but that does not matter. I am really doing it for me as well as for them. I've discovered that nothing brightens my day better than trying to brighten someone else's.

Psalm 23 "Make a joyful noise unto the Lord."

Why not to everyone else, too?

Session II

OPENING CEREMONY

Each "quitter" refers to their log and discusses any changes in her/his smoking pattern since the last meeting. Many will find that their consumption of nicotine-containing products has been greatly reduced simply because of logging the event. The habit is already being changed.

Everyone reaffirms their commitment to go to any length to complete this process. Our words have power and continuing to verbally recommit will add power to what you are doing.

Each person discusses his surprises based on the exercise in the chapter entitled "Priorities". Those who failed to do this exercise should really consider how serious they are about quitting. This program is simple but it isn't easy. It usually doesn't work for those who don't work for it; especially those who refuse to make the daily time commitment necessary for the life-style changes.

Each person reads the definitions of "habit" and "addiction" and briefly discusses their homework paragraphs. Please observe that we are attacking the habit before we go after the addiction.

Members share their morning and evening prayers with

the group so that others may glean additional ideas for prayer.

Group leader discusses changes to "Log it or skip it" program. In addition to time of day and current activity, we will now also log the level of desire for this cigarette rated 1 (little) to 10 (probable death without it).

This week's log will look something like this:

Monday, 4-16-2012

7:15AM after breakfast (10)

8:05 driving to work (5)

9:15 coffee break (9)

10:00 at desk (4)

10:45 getting coffee (8)

11:30 in the car going to lunch (8)

12:35 after lunch (10)

12:38 after lunch (7)

12:55 going back to work (6)

Etc.

Each quitter must change to a new brand for every purchase this week. "Lights" of your current brand or regulars of the brand of "Lights" you've been smoking are excluded. Please remember that you may only buy one pack at a time and once you've bought a particular brand, you may not buy that brand again. Keep track of the brands as you buy them to prevent recycling

Group leader explains that some may wish to quit entirely before our official quit date. I recommend that members refrain from quitting entirely until after the 4th meeting.

Leader passes out two-piece travel toothbrushes and travel-size toothpaste. These are available at any drug store.

Quitters commit to brushing their teeth at random times each day. 5 per day is a minimum (7 if you count morning and night). Occasionally just step into the nearest public bathroom and brush your teeth. Be sure to brush the roof of your mouth and your tongue also.

Leader explains the "Hard, Deep Breath" desire reduction technique and leads the class in several of them.

"Hard, Deep Breath" technique: When an urge to smoke occurs and the member decides to pass on it, he takes three very hard, very deep breaths, exhaling vigorously each time. The third exhalation is followed by physical movement such as getting up and walking into the restroom to brush his teeth or moving to another chair. In the car he can move both legs and slide his buttocks left and right a little bit.

Using this technique the quitter will rarely have an urge that lasts 30 seconds. THIS REALLY WORKS!

Practice this technique several times per day, even when you don't want a cigarette.

If time permits, see if anyone has suggested changes to the "CEREMONIES" or needs to change their meditation time. Meditation is not optional! It is one of the absolutely indispensable keys to quitting. You can make time for it if you are deadly serious about stopping smoking.

Some members who choose morning meditation will later complain that they don't have time for it in the morning or that they are too tired to do it. Their problem is probably not in the morning. It is at night. Please remember that this is a huge life-style change. Many quitters will have to change their evening rituals to make it. The need for an earlier bed time is common.

HOMEWORK

Make a graph of your number of cigarettes smoked per day. Begin with the day BEFORE our first meeting. Write a paragraph on your analysis of the data from your "log". What time/times of day did you have the strongest desire to smoke? Also, what activities seemed to be the most smoking related?

Look up the word "lung" in a dictionary and write the definition.

Read the sections in this book entitled **Spread Joy** and **Send Love**.

Our quit date is three weeks from today.

CLOSING CEREMONY

SPREAD JOY

I first acquired a Spiritual Advisor about 27 years ago. It was a very good thing for me. I hold myself accountable to him. He knows all of my secrets and I have followed his advice with much success. I have had several Spiritual Advisors over the years. Here is some of their wisdom.

Spread joy. Find ways daily to share happiness. You can't keep happiness if you don't give it away. Plus, if I spend my day sloshing joy on others there is no way to keep it from splattering onto me. Here are some of the ways I try to spread joy:

I pray each morning to treasure my spouse and that I might not miss any opportunities to serve her today.

I smile as much as I possibly can.

I'm playful in crowds, especially in elevators and in long lines. I can lighten the burdens of others if I will stay alert for ways to do so.

I say thank you as much as I can. Sometimes I am able to see someone's whole face change when I thank them. We all need to be appreciated. I especially like to thank folks who are working when I am not. The following story is how I finally got this lesson.

As I walk the spiritual path, lessons appear at unexpected times. Several years ago we ran out of milk at noon on Christmas Day so, ...at half-time, I ran out to the car, raced down to the convenience store, rushed back to the cooler and grabbed a gallon of milk.

As I hustled up to the counter I received a gift. The gift was that I saw a human standing behind the counter on Christmas Day, probably working for minimum wage time and a half. I can't explain this very well but my heart opened up to him and said out loud, "Thanks for working on Christmas Day. I bet there is somewhere you'd rather be but, you see, my family ran out of milk and if you hadn't come in today we couldn't have gotten it. Thank you for working on Christmas Day."

He and I both cried as I said this. I'm not sure what the other folks in line behind me thought but I was so glad I spotted one of The Master's Kids who deserved to be thanked and was able to thank him.

These days I travel a lot on weekends. I am careful to express thanks to restaurant and airline employees for their weekend work. Sometimes I don't think they even notice that I said it but that does not matter. I am really doing it for me as well as for them. I've discovered that nothing brightens my day better than trying to brighten someone else's.

Psalm 23 "Make a joyful noise unto the Lord."

Why not to everyone else, too?

SEND LOVE

Matthew 5: 43-44 "Ye have heard that it hath been said, Thou shalt love thy neighbor, and hate thine enemy. But I say unto you, Love your enemies, bless them that curse you, do good to them that hate you, and pray for them which despitefully use you, and persecute you…"

Some friends and I went on a retreat to a state park. We agreed to have no contact with the outside world from Friday noon until Sunday noon. No TV, radio, newspaper or phone except for incoming emergencies.

One of the concepts we were working on was given to us by a lady who had recently come out of a coma. While in the coma she reported that she could feel the prayers and love that were being sent to her. We decided based on her testimony that it was possible to send love to people who are alive and also to those who are on the other side of the Veil.

There was no light except from the fireplace. We put our chairs far enough apart so that we were not touching but close enough so we could hold hands. Since God is Love and is the Universal Source of Love, we sat quietly in His Presence for about half an hour, asking Him to fill us with His Love.

At the end of the appointed time we held hands and each in turn mentioned a person's name. The person could be alive or not. "God help us to send Love to John." As each name was mentioned, each of the others sent our love toward the speaker and he focused it and sent it on.

Frequently we named people the others didn't know. Going counter clockwise it did not become my turn until I had sent at least three breaths of love to the person on my left. This kept us from rushing it.

I imagined a column of Love about the diameter of my head, coming out of Heaven down through the top of my head and out of my chest and out of my nose and mouth as I exhale. My column is silver and shimmers. Others report gold, etc.

We did this for about half an hour. We closed with more quiet time in The Master's Presence and a prayer of thanksgiving for this time.

I can't say what affect our sending love in what we now call The Love Meditation had on those to whom we sent love. I can tell you that the effect on those of us who participated in it defies description.

I understand that God is Love. When we give love we give God. It is as simple as that.

Before I get out of bed, I like to send love to every place I will visit during the day, and to every person I will see. I imagine a round stream of love shooting out of Heaven, down through the top of my head and out my chest. It rushes to the places I send it.

I always set 2 alarms, usually 10 to 20 minutes apart. The second one is set for the time I plan to arise. When the first sounds, my wife and I cuddle and say our morning prayers in each other's arms. I include the sending of love to the places and people in this prayer session.

I also send love to the places my wife will go that day and send healing love to anyone I know who is in need.

I spend a few moments in my car sending love into each place I am about to go and especially to the specific individuals I expect to see there.

Several years ago I had a life changing experience with this concept. I was a multi-line manufacturer's representative and had an assistant named Sheila. Sheila was a fine, Christian woman of high moral character and an excellent worker.

Our biggest manufacturing client was controlled by a woman who was extremely difficult to deal with. She was a problem for us almost every day and was well known in my industry as a major pain. Most of the reps I knew around the county were certain there was a broom in their parking lot somewhere. I said she had been that way since that house fell on her sister.

One morning Sheila and I were talking about this woman in very derogatory terms as we started our day. Sheila paused for a moment and thought and then said, "Neither of us believes we are supposed to be talking bad about anyone. We need to stop it."

She was right. I proposed that we not only stop at once but we begin every business day sending this woman love for 5 minutes. Sheila agreed. That was on a Monday or a Tuesday. By Friday of that same week the problem woman had begun to call our office just to chat. In less than a week she became our easiest factory person to deal with and remained that way.

A few months later I attend an industry trade show in

Chicago. I walked into a large meeting room this factory had secured for a hospitality party and this problem woman charged across the room, knocking people out of her way to get to me. She gave me a big hug and told me that I was her favorite rep and if she had more folks like Sheila and me to deal with her life would be so much better.

For the balance of the evening everyone who I talked to wanted to know how I had swung the wicked witch to my side. There were few people who I saw for the next few days at the show who did not ask the same question. I always gave them the same answer, "I'll tell you but you aren't going to believe it. We send her a bunch of love every morning."

I am sad to report that I don't think any of them believed me. A few months later this lady took a job with another firm and had no business reason to continue to contact us. We continued to hear from her several times a month for the next few years.

A friend of mine writes TV shows. He had a personality problem with his producer and I gave him the magic formula of sending love. He started at once. A few days later he was on a coffee break, sitting in his car talking to me on his cell phone. I heard a tapping sound and he said, "Please hold for a minute."

I heard his window go down and heard his and a woman's voices. Then I heard his window go up. He said, "UNBE-LIEVEABLE! It's raining here. That was my producer. She is going out to one of those fancy coffee shops and wondered if she could bring me a coffee and a sweet roll. Sending love really works!"

Matthew 6: 1-4 "Take heed that ye do not your alms before men, to be seen of them: otherwise ye have no reward of your Father which is in heaven. Therefore when thou doest thine alms, do not sound a trumpet before thee, as the hypocrites do in the synagogues and in the streets, that they may have glory of men. They have their reward. But when thou doest alms, let not thy left hand know what thy right hand doeth. That thine alms may be in secret: and thy Father which seeth in secret himself shall reward thee openly."

Session III

OPENING CEREMONY

Each "quitter" refers to his log and discusses any changes in his/her smoking habit since the last meeting and reaffirms their commitment to go to any length to complete this process.

Write down any patterns you can find. For example, is the cigarette with morning coffee a 9 or 10 on the need scale? How about the one after lunch?

Be sure to pay close attention to the time and related activity of your 8's, 9's and 10's. These will probably require extra attention later.

"Quitters" discuss the sections on **Spread Joy** and **Send Love** and talk about how they can incorporate these into their day. Several also read their definitions of lung.

Leader discusses changes to "Log it or skip it" program. Continue to log time of day; current activity; level of desire for this cigarette rated 1 (little) to 10 (probable death without it).

We will now also log how good/satisfying the cigarette was on a scale from 1 (not good) to 10 (WOW!). This portion of the log is completed after the cigarette has been extinguished.

Your log will typically look something like this:

Monday, 4-23-2012

7:15AM after breakfast (10) (10)

9:15 coffee break (9) (7)

10:45 getting coffee (8) (9)

11:30 in the car going to lunch (8) (8)

12:35 after lunch (10) (10)

12:55 going back to work (6) (5)

Etc.

Note that several of the times where a cigarette was logged last Monday are not logged here. That is because by now you will probably be skipping the "less than 5" urge smokes by using the hard, deep breath technique.

The facilitator explains the brand change program. Those who have been smoking unfiltered cigarettes (Camels, Pall Mall, etc.) now must buy filtered. Those who have been smoking filters

(Marlboro, Winston, etc., including "Lights") must now change to menthol filters. Those who have been smoking menthols (Salem, Kools, etc.) must now change to non-menthol filters.

Everyone must change brands with every purchase and no alternating or going back to a brand you've already bought during this process.

We will continue to "log" all cigarettes and study all data collected to determine patterns.

Each "quitter" agrees not to use any alcohol or any drugs

not prescribed by a doctor for the next 60 days. "Not any" means none at all! This is a critical commitment.

Alcohol and drugs decrease inhibitions and make smoking cessation extremely difficult. Those who are unable or unwilling to stop alcohol and drugs for this brief period are probably in some stage of addiction and should be counseled accordingly but not excluded from the group.

Continue to brush your teeth at least 5 random times per day.

HOMEWORK

Write the answers to the following questions:

1. What time or times of day do you have the strongest cravings?
2. What activities are the most smoking related for you?
3. What time and activity produce the most satisfying smoke?
4. What can you do instead of that activity that is not smoking related or what can you do IMMEDIATELY before or after that activity to help reduce your hunger for a smoke?

Change "CEREMONIES" and meditation times as needed.

Start exercising. Start slowly if you have not been exercising all along. See your doctor first if you have even the slightest concern about this.

Walking is a great way to start. If you have been a regular

exerciser, play tennis, swim, etc., as you like but get it going.

We quit 2 weeks from today.

HOMEWORK:

Read the sections in this book entitled **Anonymous Giving** and **Forgive Them All**.

CLOSING CEREMONY

ANONYMOUS GIVING

All of my life I have been a "taker". To walk the Spiritual Walk I had to learn to be a "receiver". A receiver is very different from a taker.

To be a receiver there must be a "giver". The giver willingly imparts his gifts to the receiver. The receiver humbly receives. To do so he must admit that he would like to receive.

This is one of the Eternal Truths. "I don't know everything. I'm not supposed to."

To grasp Eternal Truths I had to first release the old baby elephant beliefs that I thought were truths. Beliefs like: never apologize, it is a sign of weakness; never surrender or quit; never ask for help; never ask stupid questions; if I can get what I want it will make me happy. None of these old beliefs turned out to be true.

Another Eternal Truth is that some of what I know for sure and certain is actually incorrect. It is my willingness to continue to search for false beliefs within me that keeps me teachable. I wonder how many other false beliefs I'm still holding on to.

Once I had been a receiver for a while, my Spiritual Advisor said that it was ok for me to begin to try to be a giver.

Takers can't be givers. What they have is not really theirs and they only give so that they may get. They barter or negotiate. They do not give. Givers are not seeking a return from the receiver. Their reward comes from The Great Giver. He blesses their hearts and lives with an inner peace and joy.

Takers do not experience this peace and joy no matter how much they are able to get back from their giving. They lack the giver's most important quality of humility.

It is humility that reminds the giver that the gifts he gives are not really his. They are gifts from The Great Giver that He is just passing on. It is this remembering that brings the joy of humility to giving.

Matthew 6: 1-4 "1 Take heed that ye do not your alms before men, to be seen of them: otherwise ye have no reward of your Father which is in heaven.

2 Therefore when thou doest thine alms, do not sound a trumpet before thee, as the hypocrites do in the synagogues and in the streets, that they may have glory of men. Verily I say unto you. They have their reward.

3 But when thou doest alms, let not thy left had know what thy right hand doeth:

4 That thine alms may be in secret: and thy Father which seeth in secret himself shall reward thee openly."

My experience is that if I do something good for someone else and no one finds out about it; God gets the credit and I get a gift. The gift is a piece of sunshine about the size of a golf ball that lodges itself in my chest. I can think about what I did at any time of the day or night and that golf ball will glow and send light throughout my whole body.

Many years ago I had an occasion to do this for the first time. It was a marvelous experience! Over the next few months I spent many hours thinking of my good deed and enjoying the sunshine transfusion that I always got from thinking about it. I never told a soul…for about 6 months. When I told, the piece of sunshine came out with my words and has not returned. This is what happened.

I walked into my first sales call and had not even put my briefcase down when the receptionist told me to go on into the buyer's office. He said he did not have time to talk today and handed me a nice order. It went that way all morning and I realized that I had had a very good week by noon and it was only Monday.

I had no other business I could do that day so I headed for a State Park to fish. There was a family having a picnic and they had a 7 year old boy. It soon became apparent that I was going to do the casting and he was going to do everything else. It was his first fishing experience and he was hooked. At 7, I had been just like him. We caught several and I spent a few minutes meeting his family.

I was at a time in my life where I had a lot of spare time so I took him on several short fishing trips just to be sure he really was a fisherman. He was.

Just after his 8th birthday he and I launched a canoe on the Buffalo River about an hour west of Nashville. We floated 5 miles in about 10 hours and caught over a hundred fish. It was one of those rare, magical days.

About a mile from the take out I heard the first clap of thunder and suddenly realized that the sky was rapidly darkening. We were really going to get it and there was nowhere to get out of the river for at least a mile. I pulled over to the side of the river under some overhanging branches and started to give God a little piece of my mind, "Can't you see Saint Scott down here taking a boy fishing!!!!!? And you have to send a *&%#* thunderstorm now!!!!!? What's wrong with YOU!!!!!?"

Fortunately I did this insanity silently. About that time this beautiful boy looked over his shoulder at me and said, "Is it ok to fish here?"

I never know when I am going to get one of these amazing lessons. This one came from a little boy while I was angry with God and was once again telling Him how to do His Job.

I have asked God to run my life any way He sees fit… no matter what. The problem is that I forget I did that. When the skies of my life blacken and I hear the thunder and know there is no way out; I think I am supposed to ask my Father the same question the little boy asked me, "Father, is it ok to fish here?"

You see, I offered myself totally to God. Therefore the rest of my life is none of my business. The problem is that I tend to forget this and need to be reminded frequently.

I'd like to go back to the topic of anonymous giving for a moment. I know folks who are chuck full of those sunshine golf balls. You can see some of the light shining from their eyes.

Happy people sell more stuff. Others want to be around them and one way to have happy folks around you is to buy from them. Getting and staying happy is one of the keys to the vault if you sell for a living which I do.

Giving is a funny thing. You can't give without receiving and you can't receive without giving. It has never been done.

I think I finally understand my mission. I am a fisher of men.

Here are some ideas on giving anonymously:

Put some change into an expired parking meter on a stranger's car.

Drop some change near a bus stop. Generally the folks riding the bus are not doing too well financially. A stranger riding the bus might get a real lift from finding a small amount of money.

In my part of the country if you find a penny heads up it is a lucky penny and you pick it up. Don't just pass over the heads up pennies. Stoop over and turn the tails up ones to heads up so someone you will never see will get a lucky one.

Let everyone who puts on a blinker near you in traffic in. Thank everyone you can for everything they do for you. Compliment everyone you can as often as you can. The compliments must be genuine.

Pass up the really good, close in parking place especially in bad weather. Leave it for someone you will never meet so they can have the joy of finding it.

According to DR William Glasser in his book *Reality Therapy* there is an innate human need to do something that matters. I believe he is correct and anonymous giving is one of the ways I fill this basic need in myself.

FORGIVE THEM ALL

Matthew 7: 1-2 "Judge not that ye be not judged. For with what judgment ye judge, ye shall be judged: and with what measure ye mete, it shall be measured to you again."

Matthew 6:12 "Forgive us our trespasses as we forgive those who trespass against us."

Matthew 5: 43-44 "Ye have heard that it hath been said, Thou shalt love thy neighbor, and hate thine enemy. But I say unto you, Love your enemies, bless them that curse you, do good to them that hate you, and pray for them which despitefully use you, and persecute you…"

To live a spiritual way I have to be willing to forgive everyone…..EVERYONE no matter what they have done! I do NOT have to approve of what they did to forgive them.

My spiritual advisor said, "What you really want is mercy for you and justice for everyone else. It looks to me like the package God is presenting here is mercy for everyone OR justice for everyone and you are part of everyone and you get to choose."

He was right and I had been making the wrong choice for a long time. Now my problem is how can I forgive them. I try with all of my might and just can't do it. If I think about someone who has wronged me for long enough; I just start to hate them again.

Here are the simple steps he showed me that led me to

forgiving all of them.

1. Make a list of everyone that has ever made you angry.......EVERYONE...EVER.

2. Write a short summary of what they did. "Short" is the key word. He limited me to a couple of sentences.

3. Bring to mind the 3 or 4 worst things you ever did.

4.Observe that you were, by your own will, cut off from God when you did those things, i.e. if you had been living with your mind on spiritual things you would probably not have done those things. If you had been walking with God, you would have probably not even thought of doing them.

5. Begin a prayer session by talking to God about the 4 or 5 worst things you ever did and telling Him how much you crave His Forgiveness. This will put you in a very good frame of spirit.

6. Next, observe that you didn't set out to harm any of the folks you injured. I was amazed to find that this was true.

Up to here I have been acting as the prosecuting attorney at these people's trial. I had the name of the perpetrator and the exact details on their crime. That is about to change.

7. Mentally cross the courtroom and sit at the defense table. Observe that if you had had the childhood this person had; if you had the education or lack of that he had; if you had the parents he had; the hard knocks he had; the psychological problems he had; the life failures he had that you on your worst spiritual bad hair day might have done what he did. Ask God to help you with this.

8. Here is the hard part. Ask in prayer that everything

you want for yourself be given to him. Please note:

I did not ask you to mean it, simply to pray it. The prayer might sound something like this: "God I ask that this guy's hair doesn't fall out; that he gets promoted at work; that he wins the lottery; that his children go to school on scholarship and don't give him any trouble; that all of his sins are forgiven and that he walks in The Sunlight of Your Spirit constantly; that his wife is a fabulous wife; that his lawn grows lush and green but grows so slowly that he only has to mow it once a year."

Be creative! The more creative you are the better. When you finish ask yourself, "Do I mean that prayer?" This is not an essay question. It is a yes or no question. If you mean it, put a check mark by the name and go on to the next name. If you don't mean it, go on to the next name anyway.

Once you reach the end of the list, go back to the beginning and continue praying the list but only the ones that do not yet have a check mark. Do this until they are all checked.

I like to think of resentment as ice around my heart. The ice has a thickness maybe based on the severity of the offence, how long ago it happened and how much I have nurtured this old anger.

Using this method I am really holding the icy heart up to the Sunlight of the Spirit. Sunlight will melt ice but sometimes it takes a while.

I recommend regularly scheduled prayer sessions that always open with the few minutes talking to God about the 4 or 5 worst things you ever did; and telling Him how much you crave His Forgiveness; then proceed with praying for the other person as explained in 8 above.

I was amazed that eventually I began to mean the prayer for these people, one at a time. My list of about 160 names was down to around 5 within 60 days. These last 5 lingered for quite a while but eventually were and are gone. Amazing!

As I completed this process people around me saw a difference in me. I was frequently asked if I had lost weight or just received some good news. The truth is that I had lost some weight. I had lost the weight of hating some of God's Children. I had received some good news. The news was that I no longer judged them.

I believe this process is just slightly more important than life or death. In The Lord's Prayer, Jesus teaches us to say"… forgive us our trespasses as we forgive those who trespass against us…" If I understand this phrase it says, "God, if I don't forgive them, don't You forgive me." I am asking to be graded by my own standards.

I am not now nor do I ever expect to be in a position to face justice. For that reason I have chosen mercy for everyone. It has been this prayer process that has changed me the most.

The word resent comes from the Latin. "re" prefix means again; like reread or rethink. The Latin verb sentire means to feel. In English resent means to re-feel old anger.

I don't think it matters how long the process takes. What is important is that I stay in the process until it is complete.

Matthew 7: 1-2 "Judge not that ye be not judged. For with what judgment ye judge, ye shall be judged: and with what measure ye mete, it shall be measured to you again."

Matthew 6:12 "Forgive us our trespasses as we forgive those who trespass against us."

Matthew 5: 43-44 "Ye have heard that it hath been said, Thou shalt love thy neighbor, and hate thine enemy. But I say unto you, Love your enemies, bless them that curse you, do good to them that hate you, and pray for them which despitefully use you, and persecute you…"

Session IV

OPENING CEREMONY

Each "quitter" discusses any changes is her/his smoking habit since the last meeting and reaffirms their commitment to go to any length to complete this process.

Your patterns should have become pretty clear by now. Write them down.

Each "quitter" discusses the homework assignment of reading the sections in this book entitled **Anonymous Giving** and **Forgive Them All**.

They also answer the 4 questions and explain their exercise program for the past week.

Each identifies his/her own most critical smoking times and activities. They also discuss what they can do instead. Many quitters find that the cigarettes immediately following meals are the most craved and the most satisfying. Swallowing the last bite and then immediately getting up from the table and doing something can help tremendously at these times. Brushing teeth immediately following meals helps too, as does the hard, deep breath technique.

Many have found that coffee drinking is extremely triggering and have quit coffee for a few months to aid in smoking cessation. Other group members may have helpful suggestions if an individual has a particularly strong smoking related activity or time. Let's talk about it. This is a team sport!

"Log it or skip it" program continues unchanged except those who had originally smoked 'straights' now change from filters to menthol filters. Continue to buy single packs only.

Your log will typically look something like this:

Monday, 4-30-2102

7:15AM after breakfast (10) (10)

9:15 coffee break (9) (7)

10:45 getting coffee (8) (9)

12:35 after lunch (10) (10)

Etc.

Several more times and activities will probably have dropped from your log by now.

Each "quitter" will stop carrying matches, lighters or any other means of lighting a cigarette. The lighter in their automobile will be removed today. You will have to bum a light now.

Bring all smoking paraphernalia to the next meeting. This includes ashtrays, lighters, remaining cigarettes, pipes, cigars, nicotine gum, patches and any other smoking related items. Also bring mints, chewing gum, toothpicks, toothbrush and toothpaste and any other non- tobacco "busy hands and mouth" goodies you can think of.

HOMEWORK: Look up the words "withdrawal" and "meditation" and write the definitions.

Fill in the following mathematical blanks: 85 minus _________(your age) = _________ X 365 X ______ (# of cigarettes per day you were smoking the day before our first meeting) =_________________ = The approximate number of cigarettes you would have smoked in your lifetime if you didn't quit now. Bring this math to the next meeting.

Example: You are 40 years old and smoked 1 pack per day before you started this program:

85years minus 40 years=45 years X 365 days= 16425days X 20 cigarettes per day

=328,500 cigarettes you would have smoked from now to age 85

This is a BIG NUMBER don't quit them all at once. When you quit, only quit for those cigarettes of that day. That number is much easier to deal with.

Read the sections in this book entitled **Today** and **The Last Right Thing**.

Our quit date is one week from today.

CLOSING CEREMONY

TODAY

Matthew 6:31 "Therefore take no thought, saying What shall we eat? Or, What shall we drink? Or, Wherewithal shall we be clothed?

Matthew 6:34 "Take therefore no thought for the morrow: for the morrow shall take thought for the things of itself. Sufficient unto the day is the evil thereof."

One of the most difficult concepts I have ever tried to apply to my life is "one day at a time". It means I should stay in this day not only physically but also mentally and spiritually.

An important sub-concept is not to borrow pain or pleasure from the past or from the future. I am more guilty of borrowing pain. I say things to myself like, "This has been going on for sooooo long;" or "How much longer do I have to endure this." These are common examples of borrowing pain from other days.

The Master said, "Take no thought of the morrow, of what you will wear or eat. The troubles of this day are sufficient." Matthew 6:34

This does not mean that I don't plan future actions as part of today's assignment. It means I don't figure out all of the "what if's" that go with it. I book hotel rooms and schedule appointments with customers. I don't figure out what the customer is going to say and then what I'll say and then what he'll say…ad nauseum.

I plan action. This is part of an orderly, spiritual life and is healthy.

If I project results it means I'm getting out of today and that is unhealthy.

Planning makes me more efficient. Projection makes me crazy and saps my strength. I only get a certain amount of spiritual energy each day. If I squander it on things over which I have no power, I will not have enough left to handle the things that are truly mine to handle today.

One of my mentors used to say, "It is like God and I are on a tandem bicycle. He is up front steering. I am in the back peddling. I can steer anytime I want but He won't peddle." Any time I get off into the future trying to figure it all out, I am trying to steer.

According to the Bible, Moses and the Israelites were fleeing Egypt with the Pharaoh's army in hot pursuit. Moses knew the geography of the region and was aware that they were headed for the Red Sea. He also knew there were no boats, no bridges and no hope of circumnavigating the Red Sea in the time available.

What was Moses real job in light of these circumstances? His job was to try to get his sandals wet. He needed to do all he could and leave the rest to God. Not to worry or to wring his hands because of his eminent demise or even to expect a miracle one minute before it was needed. His job was to have and demonstrate faith.

How do I try to get my sandals wet? I do it by staying in the day and doing all I can, leaving the rest to Him.

I like to use the word "today" as much as I can in my

speech but also in my thoughts and prayers. This helps me to hold focus and greatly increases my efficiency. As an old friend of mine says, "Wherever you're at, be there!"

When I find I am having trouble staying in today, I make some signs about 7" square that say, "TODAY" in dark magic marker. I put one on top of my sox in the sox drawer, one on top of the underwear, one on the mirror where I shave, one on the dash board of my car and one in my desk. I also cut 2 the size of a dollar bill and put one on the inside of my folding money and one on the outside and I say "Today" every time I see one.

Lack of acceptance is one of the most corrosive of all of the mental problems. Acceptance does NOT have to include approval. Acceptance is when I stop fighting, on a heart level, something over which I have no power. Some examples are the actions of bosses or of adult children. I don't have to approve to accept. If I have power and choose not to use it, I am really surrendering when I could win.

A few years ago the 100th Psalm caught my heart's eye and I saw it as I had never seen it before. It appears to me to be the directions for starting my prayers.

"Make a joyful noise unto the Lord…Come before his presence with singing…Enter into his gates with thanksgiving and into His courts with praise, be thankful to Him…"

I find that when I follow these simple instructions by opening my prayers with thanksgiving and praise, the prayers just feel better. I am convinced that all of the blocks in the channel between me and God are at my end. His end is clear. It is thanksgiving and praise that seem to clear the blocks for me.

I open my prayers with thanks per the 100th Psalm. Then I invite God in to run my life today. I especially ask Him to open me to His Guidance and to not let me miss a single opportunity to be of service to Him or to any of His Children today. I ask him to make me a great husband to my wife, a great father to our children, a wonderful grandfather to the grandchildren and a great employee today. I also ask Him to help me to send love to all of the places I plan to go this day, one at a time; and to help me send love to any persons who vex my spirit or who seem to me to be in need of healing or guidance. I also like to send love to those who have decided to attack my country and to be our enemies and I invite Him to change my plans any way He sees fit. I thank Him for my family and for the wonderful life I have been given.

Usually, after these prayers, I shower and meet my wife on the sofa where we read from spiritual literature and meditate from 5 to 20 minutes.

I close my day with thanks for the day and a review of the events of the day and inquire if I have left anything undone or if I need to repair any damage I may have done this day. I offer God the night and ask Him to govern my dreams. Occasionally, after the lights are out I will send love to individuals. It is a fine way to close the day.

THE LAST RIGHT THING

Some of us are fond of saying that we are only responsible for doing the "next right thing". I like the idea. It leaves God in charge of long range plans and goals and leaves me in charge of action in the moment.

Recently I discovered that there is a "last right thing". The last right thing for me is to go to bed at a reasonable hour and set an alarm. My bedtime must be a time which will assure that I can get sufficient rest and be able to arise early enough to have plenty of time in the morning to begin my day with prayer, reading and meditation. My morning routine usually takes me about half an hour. If I fail to do the last right thing tonight I won't be able to do the first right thing tomorrow.

Session V

OPENING CEREMONY

Each "quitter" discusses any changes to his/her smoking pattern since the last meeting and reaffirms their commitment to go to any lengths to complete this process.

Everyone tells the group their math homework.

Leader initiates a trashcan ceremony and each quitter throws away all ashtrays, lighters, cigarettes, etc,. with the statement. "I AM NOW A NON-SMOKER!"

Remember! "One puff is too many and 1000 were never enough!"

Several members read their definitions of withdrawal and meditation.

The group discusses the sections in this book entitled **Today** and **The Last Right Thing**.

The leader re-emphasizes the "one day at a time" concept and reminds everyone to ask in morning prayer for the strength to not smoke just for today. The leader also reminds everyone of the importance of not discussing this program with anyone for the next 60 days. Don't even tell your best friend you are quitting. You don't want to set yourself up for a friend to approach you at a time when you aren't even thinking about a smoke and say, "How are you doing on that quit smoking thingy."

Each "quitter" discusses her/his own most difficult times and activities; what they are going to do to win at those times; and verbally commits to those behaviors in front of the group.

Each "quitter" practices saying, "I'm just not smoking today", and "I don't want to talk about it". These are the answers to friends' questions and will be needed. Practicing in group will help a lot.

Each "quitter" recommits to go into the nearest washroom and brush her/his teeth AT LEAST 5 times a day. Discusses the appropriate times for the use of mints, toothpicks, etc. Sometimes just holding a pen in one hand can be helpful.

HOMEWORK:

Fill in the following mathematical blanks: 85 minus _____ (your age) X 365 X _____ (number of packs you were smoking per day the day before our first session. Include partial packs. Your number might be 1.5 packs or 2.2) X $______ (the price per pack today) =$ ________ This is the amount of money you would have spent in your lifetime on cigarettes if you didn't quit (assuming the price doesn't go up, HA!)

Example: You are 40 years old and smoke 1.5 packs per day at $5.00 per pack

85 years – 40 years = 45 years X 365 days = 16424 days X $7.50 = $123,180 you will save to age 85 if you quit now.

Read the section in this book entitled **Dream Big.**

CLOSING CEREMONY

DREAM BIG!

I had the privilege of flying for the United States Air Force for 5 years in my early 20's. The T-38 Talon was a brand new high performance trainer, just into the inventory. The single seat version is the F-5 which is still in use around the world as a super-sonic interceptor.

My last flight in the T-38 I did a "burner climb" to 40,000 feet. It took 3 and ½ minutes from break release on the runway to get to 40, 000 feet. Jacksonville Center gave me a 30 mile circle around a point on the ground and an altitude block that would contain no other aircraft while I was there. You need a lot of room if you're going to play at 9/10ths of the speed of sound which is around 700 miles per hour.

The altitude block they gave me was from 18 to 60 thousand feet. Our instructors warned us on a weekly basis not to go above 45, 000. The air is so thin above 45 that things can happen from which you will not recover.

In 1967 the radar did not give the controller your altitude or airspeed as it does today and I was young and immortal. I eased the throttles back out of afterburner as the T-38 afterburner uses fuel so fast that you can actually see the needles on the gas gauges move. I rolled her into about 15 degrees of right bank to keep me in my 30-mile circle and let her climb.

10 miles of altitude would have been 52,800 and I

thought I was going to make it but at 52,300 she was done. I was traveling at 9/10ths of the speed of sound using all of the power available short of afterburner and my climb was over.

I had done what is known as an instrument climb which means that I had been looking at my gauges and had not looked outside. When she quit climbing I rolled out on a northerly heading and looked up. I was about 80 miles west of Jacksonville, Florida out over the Okefenokee Swamp. It was about 9:30 on a clear morning and a bright sun was coming up over my right shoulder. Straight up through the bubble canopy the sky was jet black. I looked out to the west and saw the curvature of the Earth and I don't mean a little bit. The horizon was curved forward and aft of my craft.

I had a sensation like someone was pouring something warm over my head and it was running down over my body like wax running down the sides of a candle. I suppose it was a lot like being anointed. At the same time I was overwhelmed by a peace like I had never known. I felt like I was looking at eternity.

This planet we are riding is just a big blue ball, floating in space, held there by love I guess. I didn't see anything else.

In the poem *High Flight* the author says, "I put out my hand and touched the face of God." I understand that now. I touched The Master's Face that day.

I sat there for only a couple of minutes in awe and then gently reduced the throttles and slowly descended to land. I couldn't tell anyone because I would be in big trouble if any of my superiors found out.

For over 25 years I have wanted to see the curvature of

the Earth again. I don't suppose it is possible to do something like that and not want to do it again.

In 2004 my little business had a pretty good year. My bride and I charted a Leer 31. My pilot's license isn't current so they won't let me sit in the front row any more so we also chartered 2 pilots from a local air charter service. A Leer 31 will go to 51,000 and this one did.

One of the hardest things for me to learn has been to dream big. I serve a Big God Who wants all kinds of great things for me. I need to expect miracles and joy and love and freedom and I plan to see the curvature of the Earth again. Don't you?

I am learning to Dream Big! It is my hope and prayer that this book will help you to drop some of your baby elephant beliefs and to begin to Dream Big.

Session VI

OPENING CEREMONY

Each "quitter" discusses his/her success or problems honestly and asks for group support. Discuss any new ideas that may help others stay quit. Discusses her/his most difficult times and verbally recommits to the substitute behaviors previously selected. Announces their number of tooth brushings per day.

Group members share their math homework and discuss the section entitled **Dream Big**.

The leader breaks the group into teams with two, three or four quitters on each team. Team members are responsible for communicating with every team member every day until the next session. Try to limit your team discussion of quitting to new ways you have found that help and thanks for others being there for you.

A group member leads group meditation.

Continue to refrain from telling ANYONE you are quitting smoking.

1. You're not quitting. You are now a non-smoker.

2. You don't want anyone reminding you of smoking by asking about it.

3. You don't want to squander your "clean lung energy" talking about something that is not a "clean lung" subject.

4. If someone presses you, say, "I'm just not smoking today." If you're really doing "one day at a time" this is true.

5. Continue the random tooth brushing at least 5 times per day.

6. Continue meditation at least 15 minutes per day. Team members or group members may decide to meditate together. Good Idea!

7. Continue the "hard deep breath" technique anytime you get an urge.

8. Continue with morning prayer for help this day.

9. Continue a regular exercise program with your doctor's approval.

HOMEWORK:

_______ (number of packs per day you smoked before our first session) X 365 X _______ (Price per pack) = $_______ per year you spent on smoking.

Ask a banker what that amount added every year to a compound interest account would be worth in 80 minus _______(your age) years. Bring that number to the next session.

Example: You are 40 years old and smoke 1.5 packs per day at $5.00 per pack. 1.5 packs X 365 days = 547.5 packs per year X $5.00 = $2737.50 per year cost.

Assuming you quit now and deposit your cigarette money annually in a bank at 3% compound interest for 45 years, ignoring inflation, your total on hand will be $253,820!

Please be sure you are making all of the necessary life style changes. YOU ARE NOT FINISHED! CONTINUE TO MEET WEEKLY FOR SUPPORT!

CLOSING CEREMONY

HOW TO CRY

I believe that my emotions are the channel my Spirit uses to communicate with my Mind and my Body. If I block any of that channel, I block all of it to some extent.

I always thought that crying and laughing were opposites. They are not. They are siblings. Both are involuntary emotional releases. Since I learned to cry my laughter comes from a different place, deeper in my spirit. My tears come from that same place. It was necessary for me to learn to feel my feelings so I could touch that place. It is a gentle place of feeling.

Crying and laughing are also similar physically. When I laugh my stomach muscles flex and relax my face flushes red and my breathing takes on an irregular pattern. When I cry all of these occur, too.

I learned as a child to stop the flow of tears by hearing my father scream, **"If you don't stop that crying, I'll give you something to cry about**!" I learned to stop the tears by flexing the muscles that surround my tear ducts. I did it so often that I forgot how to relax them.

I didn't really need to <u>learn</u> to cry. I needed to <u>unlearn</u> not to cry.

I had also learned not to focus my mind on anything that would evoke my emotions to a point that I might begin to cry. I needed to re-learn/remember how to stay in a mental place of feeling.

Anything worth doing is worth doing poorly as I learn

to do it. One of the most important things I learned was not to expect instant success. I learned not to beat myself up for being unable to cry. I believe that chastising myself for my inability to let the tears flow would have made me less able to feel. It would have strengthened my need not to feel and slowed the process considerably.

This process takes time. It took me over a year before I was able to cry the first tear. It was worth the time and effort and wait. If you can't cry you have probably been blocked for a number of years, decades in many cases. It will take time to change. Please commit the time and be patient with yourself.

I would suggest that you begin each session with a prayer. Just tell God what you are trying to do and ask for His help. Then sit quietly for a few minutes in His Presence.

There are several tools that gave me considerable assistance in my quest for tears. *The Reader's Digest* and *Chicken Soup for the Soul* contain lots of heart-warming stories in every copy. I suggest that you select a quiet spot, maybe under a tree in your back yard or by a gently flowing river or in a room in your home where you won't be interrupted. Begin to read.

When you feel the emotions starting to flow and the need to cry emerges, stop reading and focus on whatever you just read. Do not focus on trying to cry, as this will stop the emotional feelings. Think of the beautiful passage you just read and try to relax the muscles in your face and begin to flex and relax your stomach muscles. Think of the passage as long as you can and continue to try to slacken your facial muscles and flex and relax your stomach muscles. Do this until you feel the emotional peak has passed or until your tears begin to flow.

Once the emotional peak has passed, whether you cried or not, reread the passage and if you are able to touch the feelings again, repeat the process. If your urge to cry does not reappear, continue reading until you are touched again.

I suggest you plan about three sessions per week of about 30 minutes each.

Another good tool is movies. Go to "chick flicks". There are some really touching ones. Use the same physical exercises mentioned above as you feel the need to cry in the theater.

Certain books are also great tear starters. As I mentioned above all of the *Chicken Soup for the Soul books* are excellent tear starters and one of my favorite novels is *The Education of Little Tree*. Use the same technique we discussed above.

CD's are another good source of emotional food. *The Education of Little Tree* is available on CD as are a number of other books and seminars. I also suggest anything by Leo Buscalia.

My own first break through was via audio-tape. I was traveling a lot during the time I was trying to learn to cry. I would listen to tapes and when something would touch me I would try to cry.

For months I couldn't even get close. Eventually I would feel like I was about to start to cry so I would pull over to the side of the road. As soon as I put on my blinker and started to slow down the feeling would pass. This happened many times before I was able one afternoon to get the car stopped and sit still and cry. What an exhilarating experience!

It was wonderful to be able to finally get a few tears out but it was not like the dam had burst. I still had to continue to make effort and do the things we've talked about for many months to improve on my ability to let the tears flow.

Today I can cry whenever I'm moved to, but my learning is incomplete. I am now in the process of learning to talk while I cry. I have some success to report but this part of my process is not finished.

My ability to stop tears did not go away. I can stop them anytime. If I'm in an inappropriate place for crying, I delay the tears until a better time.

Once your ability to cry is relearned you may find yourself crying at times and not knowing why. Don't worry about it. Your mind doesn't have to know why you are feeling. Besides, you are probably a few decades behind on your crying. Maybe you are just catching up!

When I've had a good cry I feel like my soul has had a warm shower and dried off in the sunlight of the spirit. I hope this process blesses you as it has me!

WARNING TO MEN!

If you start crying at appropriate times and places you will attract a lot of very healthy women. Please don't contact me to complain about this. I warned you here.

Most women are just plain sick of the "John Wayne Act" so many men have been doing and they see right through it. When healthy women see a man who is in touch with his emotions it lights them up like Pinball Machines.

By the way, don't worry about attracting all of these healthy females if you are married. The healthy ones never attack a marriage. There is no "downside" to learning to cry.

TURNING BIG DEALS OVER TO GOD

I moved out of the home my first wife and I shared about six years after my White Light experience. It just wasn't working and we were both angry a good bit of the time.

I found a small apartment and set up bachelor housekeeping. I was most confused as I didn't believe in divorce but I also knew that she and I couldn't live together peacefully. There seemed to be no answer.

One evening, alone in a small apartment, I asked God for an answer. It is not my mission to convince you that what I am about to tell you came from Him but you should know that I believe it did. What I got that night was a group of three prayers and I prayed them daily for almost three years.

"If it is Your Will for us to be together, put us together."

"If it is Your Will for us to be apart, put us apart."

THOSE ARE THE EASY ONES! Here is the one that made the difference for me.

"If it is Your Will for me not to know today… leave me not knowing."

When I can pray that one and mean it, I can get my spiritual advisor's definition of serenity. He said that serenity isn't freedom from the storm. Serenity is peace in the midst of the storm. The only way I can have that peace is if I can give up my need to manage the storm. This third prayer helps me give up the need to manage.

For many years I had believed that "not knowing" was what was making me crazy. Incorrect! It was "needing to know" that was sapping my serenity. Only when I give up the need to know, can I be at peace during a "big deal". Strangely enough, when I give up the need to know, I begin to know.

That third prayer has given me that peace during a number of life's storms. If I really want only His Will then I don't need to know anything about the future except that He holds it in trust for me.

Sessions VII through XI

OPENING CEREMONY

Each "quitter" discusses his/her success or problems honestly and asks for group support. Discuss any new ideas that may help others stay quit. Discuss her/his most difficult times and verbally recommits to the substitute behaviors previously selected. Announces their number of tooth brushings per day.

Team members are responsible for communicating with every member of their team every day until the next session. Try to limit your team discussion of quitting to new ways you have found that help, how much better you feel, athletic activities, and thanks to others being there for you.

How did your team do on communication? Did you choose to meditate together? If so, share the experience with the group.

Someone leads a group meditation.

Continue to refrain from telling ANYONE you are quitting smoking.

1.   You're not quitting. You are now a non-smoker. You don't want anyone reminding you of smoking by asking about it. You don't want to squander your "clean lung energy" talking about something that is not a "clean lung" subject. If

someone presses you, say, "I'm just not smoking today." If you're really doing "one day at a time" this is true.

2.	Continue the random tooth brushing at least 5 times per day.

3.	Continue meditation at least 15 minutes per day. Team members or group members may decide to meditate together. Good Idea!

4.	Continue the "hard deep breath" technique anytime you get an urge.

5.	Continue with morning prayer for help this day.

I am told that physical withdrawal from nicotine is about 40 days and some days will be easier than others. My withdrawal period was somewhat less than 40 days. I define this period as how long it took for me to go several days without thinking of or feeling like I needed a smoke.

PLEASE continue to do all of the recommended procedures until you have been smoke free for at least 60 days. It only takes one puff for you to get re-hooked and not smoking is never going to get any easier than it is today!

Stay close to your team members. You need each other and encourage each other to continue to make all of the lifestyle changes necessary.

CLOSING CEREMONY

NOTES TO GROUP LEADERS

Good meetings start on time. Great meetings end on time. Agree on start and stop times at your first meeting. I suggest one hour for groups of six or fewer and 1.5 hours for seven to twelve. Over twelve I suggest you split into several separate groups.

Continue to emphasize "one day at a time" at every meeting. Don't allow anyone to entertain the thoughts about how hard it is going to be or how long it is going to take to get through withdrawal. Today is all that matters. Borrowing pain from the future is a bad plan.

Emphasize not talking about this program to anyone. The quitters will need to use all of their energy internally. They also don't want to have this become a topic for discussion. The more time they aren't thinking about it the better. They don't need friends bringing up the subject.

Some of your "quitters" are talkers and some are listeners. Be sure everyone gets the approximate same amount of group time.

Some may actually quit before the "quit date". Encourage them. Cover this in your early meetings. Ask them to keep the group informed. Also encourage any who quit and then start back. Remind them that maybe they probably just needed the whole process.

Some of your "quitters" may have a problem with giving

up alcohol and/or drugs for the prescribed time period. This is a sure sign that they are hooked. Try to get them help for these problems but do not eliminate them from the group for this reason.

Warn them that coffee may be a bigger problem than they think. I had to quit coffee for six months because it went so well with smoking.

Physical withdrawal is usually over by day 40 after the last puff, assuming they did not substitute nicotine gum, etc. These 40 days are a dangerous time. Smugness can lead to disaster. Encourage your "quitters" to continue to attend the meetings; brush their teeth 5 times per day; exercise per their doctor, and pray and meditate daily for at least the next 4 weeks. These life-style changes are all CRUCIAL!

At day 41 the "quitters" are actually quit. It is ok for them to discuss this program or any other aspect of their cessation with others. They may even wish to facilitate a group of their own. Encourage this. It will really increase their chances of success.

Also encourage them to stay away from alcohol, drugs and coffee for several more months. These reduce the resolve and inhibitions, and tend to lead back to cigarettes.

For those who smoke again and are unable to stop, ask the questions concerning the commitments:

Did they follow ALL of the suggestions?

Did they "log" accurately and study the results?

Did they follow their own guidelines for difficult times and activities?

Did they give up drugs and alcohol?

Did they give up coffee?

Did they discuss the process with anyone else?

Did they brush their teeth 5 times a day (7 including morning and night)?

Did they meditate daily?

Did they pray daily?

Did they practice the hard, deep breath technique?

This process requires a massive commitment to make big changes. Get the truth and help them to recommit. Also solicit group support and reemphasize "one day at a time".

Definitions:

Changes in smoking pattern. These include but are not limited to changes in the number of cigarettes smoked each day, quitting altogether, failure to follow all of the suggestions, changes in the times they smoke, etc.

Smoking Paraphernalia. This includes but is not limited to cigarettes, pipes, matches, cigarette lighters, cigars, chewing tobacco, snuff, ashtrays, etc.

"Hard, Deep Breath" technique. When an urge to smoke occurs the quitter takes three very hard, very deep breaths, exhaling vigorously each time. The third exhalation is followed by physical movement such as getting up and walking into the restroom to brush his/her teeth or moving to another chair. Using this technique the quitter will rarely have an urge that lasts 30 seconds. THIS REALLY WORKS!

May God bless your efforts on this project!

ACKNOWLEDGMENTS

I first want to thank Jesus for being my Savior. I am much in need of His Guidance, Forgiveness and Grace as I am still a sinner.

My friend and mentor, Howard Pohlenz, from whom I acquired the Baby Elephant. It has been a God-send in my life for a very long time.

Special thanks to my son Travis for his editing, to my sister Laramie for her continued support and to my daughter Melissa who has supported me so well.

Bill Karlson's advice and editing were spot on as were Barbara Eaton's.

Joe Crogan and Will Dempsey were heavily involved in keeping me on track. I appreciate their friendship and their help.

Mike Fitzpatrick was the brains on the final form.

John Edwards without whose support and advice this would have not been completed.

Deborah Ezell-Denson did the original watercolor for the cover, and Dale Goodloe finalized it to its current magnificence. Thank you both.

Thanks to Wall Street Dan Schwiehs for his friendship and for providing a wonderful place for me to work.

I would also like to give special thanks to several close friends for helping me through a very difficult time in my life. You know who you are and I cannot thank you enough.

SUGGESTED READING

The following books have had major influence on my life:

The Bible

God Calling and God at Eventide, A J Russell

The Sermon on the Mount, Emmett Fox

Embraced by the Light, Betty Eady

The Parent's Tao Te Ching, William Martin

Reality Therapy, Dr William Glasser

The Greatest Salesman in the World, Og Mandino

OTHER BOOKS BY SCOTT LEE

All Schoolhouse Earth Books are based on the premise that Earth is a school and that I got here by flunking out of somewhere else or I was expelled as a behavior problem:

<u>*Spirituality for the Religiously Challenged: Schoolhouse Earth Books Volume I.*</u> This book is a set of spiritual observations, activities and lessons on developing a fun, productive and effective spiritually based life. These easy to follow directions will bring you a new joy, no matter what your religious beliefs are. They are especially effective for those who do not have a religion or a spiritual connection at all.

Salesmen Can Go to Heaven!: Schoolhouse Earth Books Volume II: Acquire an honest spiritual approach to the world of sales. Learn to make a good living selling while remaining true to the Spiritual Principles that guide the universe. This book has been authorized to and contains a full description and history of John Steinhouse's innovative concept, The Extilliation Factor.

I Think I've Gotta Be God's Favorite Kid I was diagnosed with cancer in June of 2020. While ruminating about it one day I remembered friends who have had near death experiences saying that God and I would review every day of my life when I died. I thought, "If I could relive 7 individual days of my life, exactly as they happened, which ones are they?" I came up with 14 and it put me on a Gratitude High that has lasted to today. After writing the 14 days it occurred to me that I have known some real characters. Who are they and what have I learned from each one? That is the basis for the second section of this book. The third is simply a few lessons I've learned and some spiritual practices.

Current information can be found on my web site: ScottLeeinc.com.

If you have an original short story on any topic at all that you'd like to have us publish in one of our *Other Lies* series of books; please email it to Scott@ScottLee.com along with your contact information.

ABOUT THE AUTHOR

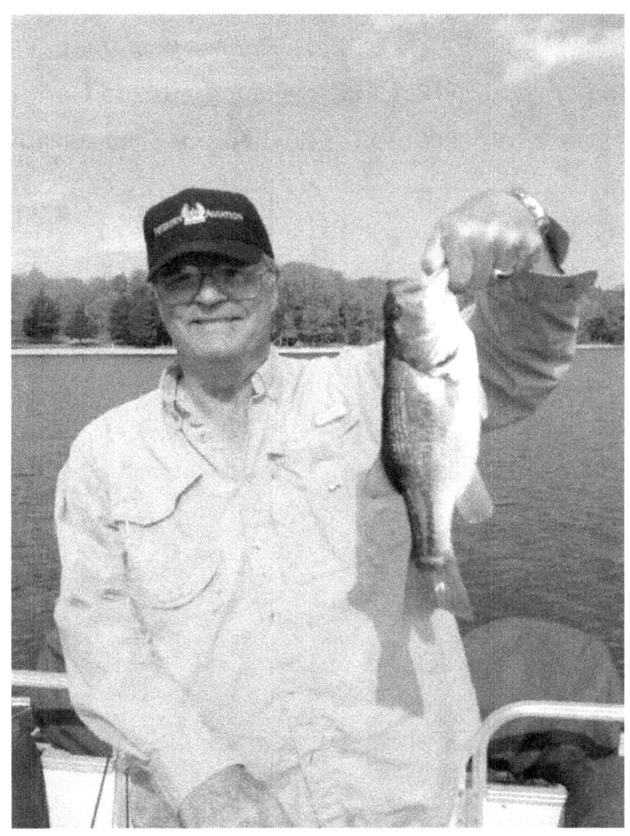

I was raised in the Presbyterian Church and am a graduate of The University of the South. I had the privilege of serving in the United States Air Force as a pilot for 5 years and was honorably discharged in 1971. I have been a Manufacturer's Representative since then.

I had a "burning bush" conversion experience in the

summer of 1984 while I was being treated for alcoholism and drug addiction and have been clean and sober since.

When I am asked what my religion is I usually say something like, "I'm trying to be a Christian." By that I mean that I believe Peter was correct, that Jesus is The Christ and that I am imperfectly following Him to the best of my willingness, probably never to the best of my ability.

One of my teachers told me that he treats God like a gentleman. Gentlemen don't go where they are not invited and they don't stay where they are not made welcome. When I awaken every morning, I invite Him into my life as Lord, Savior and Manager, not helper. Then I try to conduct myself all day long in a manner that I think will make Him welcome.

It has been my privilege to take spiritual meetings into jails, prisons and other assorted facilities for over 27 years. I'm not sure if my spiritual message has helped any of those people but I am sure that trying to carry His Message continues to help me.

The Schoolhouse Earth Books were originally my attempt to carry His Message.

NOTES

93